Content

What is Nutrisystem Diet?

Nutrisystem is a commercial weight-loss diet that involves following a meal plan made up of the company's prepackaged and portioned meals and snacks, including frozen and shelf-stable options delivered to you, complemented with some vegetables and other grocery additions you shop for yourself. By outsourcing meal-management chores, you won't have to think about portion control, meal prep or meal timing, but you may tire of heat-and-eat meals and smallish portions.

Nutrisystem says you can expect to lose up to 1 to 2 pounds per week. The program claims women can lose up to 13 pounds and 7 inches overall in your first month on the Personal Plans, and men can lose up to 18 pounds and 8 inches overall in the first month, which isn't surprising since the program makes for guaranteed calorie restriction, the tried-and-true weight-loss tactic.

Nutrisystem's high-protein weight loss plan is based on the science of the glycemic index and personal nutrition to support weight loss. With at least 75 grams of daily protein, the program is designed to keep your blood sugar steady to crush hunger and burn stubborn belly fat. It includes an all-new menu with restaurant-inspired favorites and hearty skillet dinners with more protein and vegetables included.

Nutrisystem also includes supplements, one-on-one weight-loss coaching and a mobile app for support.

Depending on your plan – there are gender-specific tracks for adults, vegetarians and people living with diabetes – you'll eat five to six times a day. There is also a partner plan designed for two people living in the same household. Most plans can be customized for those needing a lower sodium (about 1,500 mg/day) option.

Low-Calorie Diet

These diets provide far fewer calories than is generally recommended, which leads to weight loss.

Pros & Cons

Convenience of heat and eat options

No foods off-limits (not even carbs)

Eating out is limited

How does Nutrisystem Diet work?

To start Nutrisystem, you need to sign up for a specific program, select your meals and snacks from a menu (turkey sausage breakfast sandwich and flatbreads, for example) and wait for your meals and snacks to arrive. Then, if you're on the Uniquely Yours program, for instance:

The first week of your program is specially designed to jumpstart your weight loss. During this week, you'll have seven days of Nutrisystem breakfasts, lunches and dinners, seven between-meal snacks aimed at curbing cravings and keeping you feeling full, and seven shakes packed with protein to help control hunger.

After you complete your first week on the program, you'll get to create Flex Meals. That includes creating two healthy breakfasts, lunches, dinners and snacks each week so you can practice healthy cooking to help prepare you for life after being on the Nutrisystem program. In addition to the Flex Meals, the company says customers can enjoy Nutrisystem breakfasts, lunches, dinners and snacks of their choice, like a red velvet cupcake, at regular intervals, or five to six times per day.

For more support and resources, check out NuMi, a digital product for do-it-yourself dieters that integrates with wearable fitness devices and health platforms, such as the

Fitbit and Apple Health, and offers challenges to incentivize weight-loss success. Nutrisystem also runs a website called The Leaf, which provides recipes, tips on jazzing up Nutrisystem meals, fitness tips and more.

Coaches are available by phone, chat or via NuMi seven days a week (Mon-Fri 8am-10pm ET, Sat-Sun 9am-9pm ET). Those same coaches (plus Numi) can help you wean off the program once you're ready by giving your tips on how to get back in the kitchen and in front of the stove without sabotaging your weight loss.

Nutrisystem's new personalized weight-loss program takes into account a person's body type, food preferences and weight-loss goals. You'll answer some questions about yourself before checking out, and using that information, the plan is tailored to your "metabolism, age, gender, activity level and goals," according to Nutrisystem's website.

In a survey conducted among participants in a Nutrisystem-funded clinical study on the personal plans, 95% of people reported satisfaction with the variety of food, and 94% of people reported satisfaction with the structure of the program.

How does the Nutrisystem Diet Support You?

If you're looking to start the Nutrisystem diet or have already begun your dieting journey, it's helpful to know the different ways you can receive support throughout the process. Below are a few examples of how the Nutrisystem diet can support you:

As a commercial diet program, Nutrisystem offers meal delivery options that are delivered to your home.

Free assessment to determine which plan is right for you.

On demand coaching seven days a week.

The Nutrisystem app tracks your progress, provides personalized nutrition support, a grocery guide, recipes, expert tips, articles and inspiration, and weight loss challenges.

How much does Nutrisystem Diet cost?

Nutrisystem's program may be expensive or cheap, depending on what your current grocery bill looks like. The "core" four-week plan, which includes either a prepicked selection of popular foods or your choice of more than 100 foods, plus shipping, starts at around $9.29 each day on average. You can pay a few bucks more each day if you want more selection or extra protein shakes.

Remember: You've still got a monthly grocery bill to add to that. Your tab will vary depending on what produce you buy (go for anything in-season), your protein choices (chicken and turkey are generally pretty affordable) and "smart" carb choices (whole-grain pastas and beans won't break the bank).

Will Nutrisystem Diet help you lose weight?

Research – the vast majority of it company-funded – suggests you will probably lose weight on Nutrisystem. However, no new research has been conducted specifically on the Nutrisystem program in recent years.

A 2020 study published in the New England Journal of Medicine looking at the effectiveness of treatment for obesity delivered in primary care settings utilized the Nutrisystem meals as part of a "toolbox" approach for patients who were interested in using them. For patients in the intensive-lifestyle group, the weight loss goal was 10% body weight, with the initial focus of the intervention on portion-controlled foods and provision of prepackaged foods and meal-replacement shakes, including Nutrisystem meals and snacks. After the first month, patients continued to have access to Nutrisystem meals and snacks, as needed, as part of the "toolbox" approach. The study concluded "a high-intensity, lifestyle-based treatment program for obesity delivered in an underserved primary care population resulted in clinically significant weight loss at 24 months."

A 2015 study in the Annals of Internal Medicine comparing various commercial weight-loss programs found that Nutrisystem participants lost at least 3.8% more weight after three months on the program than a control group that received education and counseling. The authors call diets like Nutrisystem "promising," but say more research is needed on their long-term outcomes.

In a Nutrisystem-funded study of 69 participants with obesity and Type 2 diabetics, published in the journal Postgraduate Medicine in 2009, researchers reported that those assigned to eat meals on the Nutrisystem D diabetic track lost an average of 18 pounds after three months compared with 1 pound for the control group, who attended educational sessions on diabetes management and nutrition. At six months, the Nutrisystem dieters were down an average of 24 pounds, while the controls – who were switched to Nutrisystem meals halfway through the six-month study – were down 13 pounds.

In a similar study published in 2013 in Nutrition Diabetes, 50 Nutrisystem dieters lost an average of about 22 pounds in six months, while the 50 control dieters lost only about 5.

In another unpublished study that was funded and led by Nutrisystem, researchers reviewed self-reported weight diaries of Nutrisystem customers who were overweight or had obesity and who started the program between 2008 and 2010 and used an online tracking tool to record their weight. Data from more than 100,000 customers showed that at three months, about 79% of them had lost at least 5% of their initial weight and 33% had lost 10% or more. (Even a 5% loss can help stave off some diseases.) By six months, when 32,000 of the dieters were still recording their weight loss,

86% had lost 5% of their initial weight; 63% had lost 10 percent.

A 2013 study in the American Journal of Hypertension found that, among 41 postmenopausal women, participants on a Nutrisystem diet lost an average of 12 pounds in three months, including nearly 10 pounds of belly fat.

If Nutrisystem does encourage weight loss, it may be attributable to calorie restriction and portion control, a well-supported mechanism of weight loss. A 2013 article in the New England Journal of Medicine, for example, concluded that provision of meals and meal-replacement products promote greater weight loss than "seemingly holistic" programs based on balance, variety and moderation. While Nutrisystem once touted low-GI foods as a key element of the program, the company says it no longer claims GI to be the mechanism of weight loss.

Can you cut back on dining out? Can you withstand the temptation to eat what the rest of the family is eating most nights of the week? While Nutrisystem certainly makes dieting simple – you don't count calories, preportioned food comes right to your doorstep and you know exactly what and when to eat – you may still need to muster up willpower to stick to it.

Fortunately, you get two "flex" breakfast, lunch and dinner meals and snacks each week, which can help you keep your social engagements or answer occasional cravings. At least in the short term, you shouldn't tire of your menu choices –

Nutrisystem offers more than 160 foods to choose from on one of its most extensive plans, "Uniquely Yours Max+."

Nutrisystem is designed to be convenient. Main entrees can be ordered with the click of a mouse, but restaurant meals (and alcoholic beverages) are only occasionally allowed.

You won't need many recipes while you're on Nutrisystem, but when you do, there are simple ways to find them. If you crave a break from frozen and pantry foods, for example, Nutrisystem has a smattering of member- and company-generated recipes online, including on the website The Leaf.

Eating out is limited, but possible, on Nutrisystem. Just make sure any restaurant meal counts as one of your six "flex" meals each week. The company provides an "eating out guide" with recommendations categorized by cuisine such as

Thai, Italian and French. The guide also suggests diet-friendly foods at 30 of the most popular eateries nationwide.

Nutrisystem itself is a time-saver, since it emphasizes packaged meals. Choosing a meal plan and ordering meals is simple. While you can hand-pick each and every meal you eat, the predetermined "favorites package" is just a couple of clicks away, if you're not picky. You can also sign up for automatic billing and shipping of your food packages.

Trips to the grocery store to stock up on fresh produce, dairy and protein should be quick and can be guided by Nutrisystem's list of popular choices and recommended servings.

Nutrisystem comes with plenty of extra resources and tools. You can track your meals, exercise and weight loss online or through the NuMi app, for example; and talk with a Nutrisystem coach for support. You can even sync some wearable fitness devices with NuMi, which also acts as the official Nutrisystem tracking tool. When you're ready to wean yourself off the program, Nutrisystem offers recipes and coaches, as well as transition and maintenance plans that include a portion control container system used to make meals on your own. Online resources are free and helpful.

Hunger shouldn't be a problem on Nutrisystem. Entrees will likely be smaller than what you're used to, but you supplement them with protein, fiber-packed fruits and veggies (some even in unlimited amounts) and "smart" carbs, which generally keep you feeling fuller longer. Eating at regular intervals throughout the day should also keep tummy growls at bay.

Nutrisystem products should be palatable for most. Nutrisystem regularly introduces new items and removes items from its menu based on customer feedback, according to the company. Nutrisystem's Food and Nutrition Mission removes artificial flavors and sweeteners, colors from synthetic sources, high fructose corn syrup and artificial trans fats from its foods. The company also aims for increased transparency in its approach to ingredients.

How much should you exercise on Nutrisystem Diet?

Exercise is encouraged, but not required, on Nutrisystem. The program encourages dieters to engage in at least 30 minutes of physical activity each day, which can be broken up into three 10-minute intervals.

What types of meals should you eat on Nutrisystem Diet?

Nutrisystem takes care of dessert and your main entrees for breakfast, lunch and dinner. Depending on your plan, the choices for each might vary slightly. You can opt for only pantry items, like oatmeal, pastas and cookies, or choose a plan that includes frozen foods like omelets, chicken sandwiches and ice cream sandwiches.

Adults, people with diabetes, vegetarians and those transitioning to maintenance all have unique plans. You can't avoid the supermarket altogether, though. You'll supplement Nutrisystem meals with your favorite fresh fruits, veggies (some all-you-can-eat), lean proteins and "smart" lower-glycemic carbs.

When you wean yourself off Nutrisystem food, you can take inspiration from any cuisine to create your menu, keeping in mind the program's distinction between "good" and "bad" carbs, according to the glycemic index, a ranking of how a carb affects blood sugar levels.

Nutrisystem Diet Meal Plan

Here's a day of typical meals on a women's "Uniquely Yours" program. Nutrisystem food is noted; all other items are grocery additions, which can be substituted to suit your preferences.

Uniquely Yours Max+ Women's Plan

Breakfast

Nutrisystem buttermilk waffles.

1 cup low-fat yogurt.

Snack

2 tablespoons almonds.

1 cup strawberries.

Lunch

Nutrisystem pepperoni pizza melt.

2 cups salad topped with ½ cup chickpeas and dressing.

Snack

1 low-fat string cheese.

¼ cup whole grain crackers.

1 cup baby carrots.

Dinner

Nutrisystem hearty inspirations lemon caper chicken.

Snack

Nutrisystem ice cream sandwich.

Nutrisystem for Men

Breakfast

Nutrisystem sausage and egg muffin with 1 slice cheese.

1 cup low-fat yogurt with 1 cup berries.

1 banana.

Snack

Nutrisystem white cheddar popcorn.

1 cup baby carrots.

Lunch

Nutrisystem hamburger with lettuce and tomato

½ cup baked sweet potato fries.

1 cup sliced bell peppers.

1 string cheese.

Snack

2 tablespoons peanut butter.

1 ounce low-fat cheese.

1/4 cup whole grain crackers.

2 medium stalks celery.

Dinner

Nutrisystem sesame beef and broccoli with brown rice.

Snack

Nutrisystem chocolate chip cookies.

3-Ingredient Chocolate Pecan Caramel Bites

Ingredients:

18 pecans

6 pieces caramel chews

1 package NutriChocolaty Wafers

Directions:

Assemble pecans into bunches of 3.

Place a caramel chew on top of each pecan bunch.

Heat caramel pecans in the microwave for about 30-45 seconds, until caramels have melted.

Place NutriChocolaty Wafers in a microwave-safe bowl and microwave in 5-10 second increments to prevent burning. Continue until fully melted.

Pour the melted chocolate equally over the caramel pecans.

Allow bites to cool until chocolate and caramel harden.

Tomato and Sauerkraut Grilled Cheese Sandwich

Everyone's favorite childhood meal is made healthy and hearty with a few Extra ingredients that add major flavor. Featuring a bit of Dijon mustard, sliced tomatoes and pile of sauerkraut, our Tomato and Sauerkraut Grilled Cheese Sandwich recipe is a delicious and nutritious meal that satisfies your comfort food cravings. Find out how to make the ultimate gourmet grilled cheese in just four easy steps.

To make this easy grilled cheese, heat a pan to medium-high heat and grab two slices of seeded bread. Assemble the sandwich by spreading Dijon mustard on one slice of the bread. Next, arrange two slices of cheddar cheese on each slice of bread and lay the tomatoes and sauerkraut on the bottom slice. Close the sandwich and spread some light butter on each side. Place the sandwich on the hot pan and cook both sides until they are golden brown and the cheese becomes melted.

Enjoy your grilled cheese with a delicious bowl of tomato soup. Our Zesty Tomato Soup recipe is the perfect choice because it only contains 50 calories per serving and counts as one Extra and one Vegetable on Nutrisystem.

This Tomato and Sauerkraut Grilled Cheese Sandwich contains 394 calories. You can log it as two SmartCarbs, two PowerFuels, two Extras and half of a Vegetable in your NuMi app. Watching your carbs? Feel free to swap out the bread with a lower calorie option so that you can count it as one SmartCarb instead of two. Find a loaf of bread that provides 40 to 45 calories per slice so that two slices count as one SmartCarb. You can also substitute in your favorite type of cheese and omit the mustard if you so choose!

Looking for another creative way to cook with sauerkraut? Check out this One-Pan Simple Sausage and Sauerkraut recipe! >

Lose weight and get healthy with delicious food delivered directly to your door!

Tomato and Sauerkraut Grilled Cheese Sandwich

Ingredients:

2 slices of seeded bread (i.e. rye bread, multigrain bread)

4 ultra thin slices of cheddar cheese

1 tsp. Dijon mustard

2 slices of tomato

1/3 cup sauerkraut

2 tsp. light butter

Directions:

Heat a pan to medium-high heat.

Assemble sandwich by spreading mustard on one slice of bread. Arrange two slices of cheddar cheese on each slice of bread. Lay tomatoes and sauerkraut on bottom slice. Top with the other half of the sandwich.

Spread 1 teaspoon of butter on each side of the sandwich. Place sandwich on the hot pan.

Cook until the bread is golden brown, then flip the sandwich. Cook until the other side becomes golden brown and the cheese has melted. Serve immediately.

Low-Carb Spaghetti Squash Baked Feta Pasta

Cheesy, baked pasta dinners rarely find their way into a weight loss plan. However, if you know anything about Nutrisystem, you know that we love to take everyone's favorite meals and transform them into healthier, diet-friendly versions that don't sabotage your success. After all, the best type of diet is one that you can stick to! That's why we tasked our recipe developers with creating a lightened-up, low-carb alternative to the trendy Baked Feta Pasta that you've been seeing all over your social media feed. Featuring melty feta cheese, cherry tomatoes, olive oil and fresh basil over spaghetti squash, it's a creamy, dreamy pasta dinner that's packed with flavor.

Ingredients:

4 cups cooked spaghetti squash

2 cups cherry tomatoes

2 cups chickpeas, no salt added

2 cloves garlic, minced

1 Tbsp. olive oil

8 oz. feta cheese

2 tsp. oregano

Black pepper, to taste

¼ cup fresh basil, chopped

Directions:

Preheat oven to 400°F.

Place tomatoes, garlic and chickpeas in a baking dish. Place the block of feta in the middle. Drizzle olive oil over tomatoes and feta. Sprinkle with pepper and oregano.

Bake for 30 minutes.

Remove baking dish from the oven. Stir the mixture together. The feta should be soft and creamy.

Add cooked spaghetti squash and basil to the dish. Toss until well combined.

Chili Cheese TikTok Tortilla Wrap Hack

This TikTok tortilla wrap hack can be found all over the social media app. Users have been stuffing their tortillas with a variety of ingredients from different cuisines. Using this simple yet creative method for folding the tortillas, you can create an easy-to-eat meal that's mess-free!

Ingredients:

4 whole wheat tortillas

1 avocado, diced

1 cup turkey chili, warmed

1 cup lettuce, shredded

½ cup shredded Mexican cheese, reduced fat

Directions:

Lay a tortilla on a flat surface. Cut a slit from one side of the tortilla to the center. Turn the tortilla so that the slit is on the right side. Repeat with remaining tortillas.

Place ¼ cup of the turkey chili into the upper left quadrant of each tortilla.

Place 2 tablespoons of cheese into the upper right quadrant of each tortilla (above the slit).

Place ¼ cup of shredded lettuce into the lower left quadrant of each tortilla.

Place ¼ of the avocado in the lower right quadrant of each tortilla (below the slit).

Fold the avocado quadrant to the left over the lettuce. Then fold the tortilla up over the chili. then to the right over the cheese. You should get a triangle tortilla wrap.

Use a panini press, grill or a hot skillet to heat the wraps for 1-2 minutes per side, until lightly browned.

Air Fryer Breaded Pork Chops

Take your pork chops from "meh" to magnificent with this easy Air Fryer Breaded Pork Chops recipe! Boneless pork chops are cooked to crispy perfection in the air fryer for a hearty yet healthy dinner that tastes like you just stepped into a fancy restaurant. If you want to learn how to make thin pork chops that are crunchy, tender AND Nutrisystem-approved, read on and get cooking!

Ingredients:

1 lb. lean boneless pork chops, cut or pounded thin into 4 chops

2 eggs

¾ cup whole wheat panko breadcrumbs

¼ cup whole wheat flour

Dash of garlic powder, dried thyme, oregano and black pepper

Directions:

Preheat air fryer to 400°F.

Set up three bowls in an assembly line: Place the flour in the first bowl. Beat the eggs in the second bowl. Combine the panko breadcrumbs and seasonings in the third bowl.

Dip a pork chop into the flour to coat, followed by the eggs, then the panko mixture. (Make sure all sides of the pork chop are coated in each mixture.)

Spray air fryer basket with nonstick cooking spray. Add pork chop to the air fryer. Spray top of pork chop with nonstick cooking spray.

Cook for 6 minutes. Flip the pork chop and continue cooking for another 4-6 minutes, or until fully cooked. Repeat with remaining pork chops.

*Please note that all air fryers cook differently. Before trying any recipe, always refer to the manufacturer safety instructions provided with your specific air fryer.

Easy Slow Cooker Taco Soup with Ground Beef (High-Protein Recipe!)

This easy taco soup recipe makes six servings, so it's great for your healthy meal prep menu! One serving contains just 217 calories and counts as half of a SmartCarb, one PowerFuel and half of a Vegetable serving on the Nutrisystem program. The best part about this easy taco soup recipe? It provides a whopping 21.3 grams of protein! It's sure to keep you satisfied and energized throughout the day.

Add your favorite taco toppings to this simple and savory soup! You could even get fancy and create a taco soup bar for the whole family. Check out the list below for some topping inspiration.

Shredded Mexican cheese blend, reduced fat (2 Tbsp. = ½ PowerFuel)

Diced avocado (1 Tbsp. = 1 Extra)

Corn tortilla strips/chips (2 Tbsp. = 1 Extra)

Sour cream (1 Tbsp. = 1 Extra)

Chopped cilantro (Free Food)

Lime juice (Free Food)

Healthy Hacks: This slow cooker taco soup recipe is very versatile! Make your favorite swaps and substitutions to fit your taste buds.

Swap ground beef for ground turkey or chicken. You could even use shredded chicken!

Swap or add in your favorite spices and herbs.

Substitute black beans for white beans or pinto beans (or both!).

Use chicken or vegetable broth instead of beef broth. Swap in bone broth for even more nutrition!

Add in more non-starchy veggies like sliced bell peppers or riced cauliflower.

Ingredients:

1 lb. lean ground beef

1 onion, chopped

1 Tbsp. tomato paste

1 Tbsp. chili powder

1 tsp. cumin

1 tsp. paprika

1 tsp. oregano

1 tsp. garlic powder

¼ tsp. black pepper

1 cup corn

1 cup black beans

1- 10 oz. can fire roasted diced tomatoes

1 can fire roasted diced green chiles

3 cups beef broth, low sodium

Directions:

Heat large pan to medium-high heat. Brown the beef along with the onions.

Add tomato paste and seasonings.

Transfer mixture to a slow cooker and add the remaining ingredients.

Cover and cook on LOW for 8 hours or HIGH for 4 hours.

Dairy Free Almond Milk Eggnog

Creamy almond milk is blended to perfection by adding in delicious and savory ingredients such as honey, stevia, vanilla bean, cinnamon, nutmeg and of course, eggs! Once blended to frothy goodness, this concoction is warmed on the stove to ensure all ingredients are properly combined and settled into the mixture. The dairy free eggnog is then chilled overnight, blended again and ready to be enjoyed by the fire on a cold winter's night.

Ingredients:

2 cups unsweetened vanilla almond milk

2 eggs

1 Tbsp. honey

4-5 drops liquid stevia

1 vanilla bean, sliced in half and scraped

½ tsp. cinnamon

Pinch of nutmeg

Directions:

Combine all ingredients in a blender and blend for 60 to 90 seconds. It should look frothy.

Pour eggnog mixture into a small pot and turn heat to low. Cook for 15 to 20 minutes, making sure to stir the mixture frequently. The mixture should be warm and steaming, but not bubbling (otherwise the eggs will scramble!).

Remove the pan from the heat and allow the eggnog to cool slightly before pouring into a pitcher or jar. Chill overnight in the refrigerator to allow eggnog to thicken.

Before serving, blend again for 30 to 60 seconds if the mixture has separated.

Christmas Tree Veggie Tray

Just as colorful as it is healthy, this Christmas Tree Veggie Tray uses an array of delicious veggies to create the perfectly adorned "Christmas tree". Make a quick trip to your local grocery store to grab some cauliflower, broccoli, cherry tomatoes, bell peppers, hummus and pretzel sticks, and you are set to create the most festive (and easy) masterpiece to ever exist in the holiday realm of get-togethers. Heading to a party with a large guest list? Make two of these Christmas Tree Veggie Trays by doubling up the veggie measurements. As simple as spending a few minutes in the kitchen to cut your veggies and form your "tree," this simple snack will become your go-to food contribution for every party you attend this holiday season!

Ingredients:

3 broccoli crowns, cut into florets

1 small head of cauliflower, cut into florets

1 bell pepper, sliced thin

1 cup of cherry or grape tomatoes

1 handful of pretzel sticks

1 cup hummus

Directions:

On the bottom of a tray, place cauliflower florets to resemble snow.

Add pretzel sticks for the tree trunk.

Create tree shape with the broccoli. Add cherry tomatoes and bell pepper slices to the tree to resemble ornaments.

Top the tree with bell pepper slices crisscrossed to create a star.

Serve with hummus.

Holiday Herb Butter Roast Beef with Potatoes and Carrots

Tender, oven-roasted beef is coated in a rich and savory blend of fresh herbs and light butter, then baked to perfection with sweet carrots and hearty potatoes. Perfect for winter weather (and your weight loss plan), it's an elevated twist on meat and potatoes that you'll be craving all season!

Preparing a flavorful beef dinner with two tasty sides may seem like a lot of work. However, this dish is easy to prepare, with simple preparation and common ingredients. The roast beef and vegetables also come together in the same baking dish, which means there is one less thing to clean after the meal is done!

This recipe for Holiday Herb Butter Roast Beef with Potatoes and Carrots makes a total of 12 servings, so it works perfectly if you're having guests over for the holidays. But if you're

Christmas is a little quiet this year, that means more leftovers for you to enjoy all week.

Ingredients:

4 lb. beef top round roast, trimmed

1/3 cup fresh parsley, chopped

2 Tbsp. fresh thyme, chopped

2 Tbsp. fresh rosemary, chopped

2 tsp. minced garlic

½ onion, chopped

Black pepper, to taste

1 Tbsp. Dijon mustard

2 Tbsp. light butter

3 Tbsp. olive oil

6 cups baby potatoes

6 cups carrots, sliced

Kitchen twine

Directions:

Mix parsley, thyme, rosemary, garlic and onion together. Remove 2 tablespoons of the mixture and set it aside.

Add Dijon mustard and 1 tablespoon of olive oil to the original herb mixture and stir well.

Butterfly the roast by slicing the beef down the center and opening up the fold.

Spread the Dijon mixture over the interior of the meat. Fold it back up and tie with kitchen twine. Season the outside of the roast beef with black pepper.

Cover and let the beef rest for 4 hours.

Preheat the oven to 275°F. Place the carrots and potatoes in baking dish. Drizzle with 1 tablespoon of olive oil and season with black pepper.

Heat the remaining olive oil in a skillet set to medium-high heat. Sear the beef on all sides, until browned, about 5 minutes per side.

Transfer the beef to the baking dish with the potatoes and carrots. Bake for 1:20-1:45 hours, until meat temperature reaches 125°F.

Remove beef and place onto a cutting board. Increase the oven temperature to 400°F and continue cooking the potatoes and carrots.

Mix the remaining herb mixture that was set aside in step 1 with butter. Spread the herb butter on top of beef. Tent with foil and let rest for 30 minutes.

Slice the beef thinly and serve with cooked potatoes and carrots.

www.ingramcontent.com/pod-product-compliance
Lightning Source LLC
Chambersburg PA
CBHW051922250726

48659CB00002B/782